Chair Yoga For Seniors

The Only Chair Yoga For Seniors Program You ll Ever Need (The New You)

Daniel Mason

WHAT IS CHAIR YOGA?

Have you heard of the exceptional benefits from yoga? Of course you have. Some of the rewards of yoga include improved strength, flexibility, and overall physical (plus mental) health. You will have an immense flow of energy after yoga exercises that you and everybody else around you will notice.

Now, is it possible to do yoga from a chair?

Absolutely. You've walked a million steps and more. You've made memories that make you laugh, cry, smile and frown. And while your mind may have forgotten some details, your body has not. Your body remembers the best, warmest moments in your life. It also remembers the most challenging parts. You may think you've reached a limitation that prevents you from enjoying the rich benefits of yoga. Think again! Chair yoga places a large emphasis on foot placement. It is the foundation of your balance and mobility.

There are many yoga poses which can be modified to be performed seated comfortably. These poses increase mobility with proper breathing techniques, called pranayamas, and results in anxiety reduction and spatial awareness.

Chair yoga is an exceptional approach for older adults to get the optimal health benefits of yoga.

Is This Really Important?

As the "baby boomers" population approaches 60, the United States will face a growing problem in caring for the elderly. The younger generation is concerned about its health, however, as you've gotten older and more sedentary, you've discovered fewer methods that maintain your body, mind, and spirit in good shape.

Falls are not just the largest cause of injury related fatalities in older individuals, but they're also a major source of morbidity and disability, with head trauma, soft tissue injuries, fractures, and dislocations among the most common injuries.

Implementing chair yoga in your daily routine is extremely important. Do you suffer from chronic pain from health issues like multiple sclerosis, carpal tunnel syndrome, or osteoporosis? Have you had a hip replacement? Broken an ankle? As you reach your 60s and onward, your fitness and flexibility becomes more crucial than you might think! When suggesting chair yoga, we've heard it all. Take a look at the 3 major doubts that surround seniors embracing chair yoga.

Doubt 1: "Yoga? I can't do that, I'm too old."

Actually, regular chair yoga will boost wellbeing, empowerment, and independence. It carries low impact on the joints and improves your balance.

Doubt 2: "But I'm disabled."

Chair yoga is wonderful because it takes minimal power usage and is more accessible. You can increase blood circulation without any strenuous movements from your chair.

Doubt 3: "I'm too weak and in a lot of pain."

There are chair yoga poses specifically meant to ease back pain and arthritis symptoms. At your own appropriate pace, you can carry through each pose as comfortably as possible, and you will feel the difference with a regular routine.

There are some older adults that simply don't have time for the gym on a regular basis. Some are unable to hit the gym or classes altogether. This makes chair yoga the most effective and easily accessible alternative.

Physical Stress Improvement

As a result of stress, muscles tense up. Stress can cause muscle tension, the body's way of protecting itself from injury and pain. Muscles tense up suddenly when under sudden onset stress, and then relax when the stress passes.

Muscles in the body are in a more or less constant state of guardedness due to chronic stress. Over time, taut muscles can produce other reactions in the body, which may include stress-related disorders.

In particular, tension-type headaches and migraine headaches are frequently accompanied by chronic neck, shoulder, and head tension. Associated with stress are conditions such as low back pain and upper extremity pain, especially job-related stress.

The musculoskeletal system is responsible for causing chronic pain in millions of people. A chronic painful state is often triggered by an injury, but not always. An injured person's response to the injury determines whether or not they will suffer from chronic pain. People who maintain a certain level of moderate, doctor-supervised activity in the early stages of recovery are likely to heal faster than those who are scared of pain and re-injury and suggest a physical cause for the injury. All of these factors lead to chronic, stress-related injuries, which are related to muscle tension and eventually muscle atrophy.

Exercises, such as chair yoga, have been shown to decrease stress-induced disorders (and headaches), increase the sense of wellness, and relieve muscle tension. You'll find that muscle tension can creep into your body by any means: An unhappy thought, making mental notes, planning your next hour, etc. Any and everything can create stress in your muscles and joints.

Psychological Improvements

It should come as no surprise that yoga has mental health benefits, such as reducing anxiety and depression, since it emphasizes breathing practices and meditation. In fact, your brain might actually function better as a result.

You'll gain a sharper brain. Muscle growth and strength are the results of lifting weights. By practicing yoga, your brain cells develop new connections, and structural and functional changes take place, leading to improved cognitive skills, such as learning and memory. Memory, attention, awareness, thought, and language are just a few of the functions of the brain that yoga has an impact on. Imagine this as brain weightlifting.

According to the Sao Paulo Research Center, using MRI scans and other imaging techniques has found that regular yoga practitioners had thicker cerebral cortexes (the part of the brain responsible for processing information) and hippocampuses (the part of the brain associated with learning and memory) than non-practitioners. Yoga practitioners' brains shrink less than those who don't practice yoga, but the older ones generally shrink more. According to this study, yoga may help counteract the effects of aging on memory and cognition.

Your mood will improve. The benefits of exercise are numerous, including bringing more oxygen to your brain, lowering stress hormones, and boosting feel-good chemicals such as endorphins. However, yoga may offer additional benefits.

The limbic system, which is responsible for emotions, is also reduced during meditation. The less reactive you are, the more tempered your response to stressful situations becomes.

Traditional depression and anxiety treatments have relied on drugs and psychotherapy. Yoga is also a complementary approach that helps, and it stacks up well when compared to other complementary therapies.

Researchers reviewed 15 studies that examined the effects of relaxation on depression and anxiety in older adults in the journal Age and Mental Health. Yoga was combined with massage therapy, progressive muscle relaxation, stress management, and listening to music (we will discuss that in further detail). The most effective techniques for depression and anxiety were yoga and music. The longest-lasting effect appeared to be in yoga.

Many studies have shown that yoga is helpful for treating post-traumatic stress disorder (PTSD). By itself, it does not give relief from intrusive memories and emotional arousal, but rather as an adjunct to calming the breathing and reducing emotional arousal. The parasympathetic nervous system is activated by deep, slowing breathing, which promotes calm in people.

Trying New Things

In the beginning of your yoga journey, you probably won't be distracted as much as you're busy practicing the basic poses. When you're just learning, paying attention to your breathing is crucial, as well as learning correct posture and position. The key is to stick to the basics and not take on too much at once. Whenever you reach a more advanced level, you will be ready to learn new things and try new practices. Try to step outside your comfort zone by getting better acquainted with your yoga practice. From how your mind and body works together to understanding the energy flow and the philosophy behind it, it's natural that this may seem so fanatical.

After all, it's all new to you. When you're first starting out, you might just believe everything you hear. In order to gain an understanding of the practice of yoga, you should ask insightful questions while remaining open to all possibilities. Discovering a yoga style that is tailored to your needs begins with asking questions and trying new things.

Debunking Myths

Yoga was said to have originated in India around the year 3300-1900 BCE, though it has spread throughout the world.

Nowadays, yoga is practiced around the world, and since it's a cross-disciplinary group of mental, physical, and spiritual disciplines, it has a range of benefits to offer to everyone with an interest in living a healthy lifestyle. A lot of people believe yoga goes beyond just exercise into a way of life, and avid practitioners will tell you as much.

According to relaxation expert Mira Rekicevic of Permaculture Research Institution, the world's 55 million new yoga practitioners are expected to hit the mat in 2020, says a recent study. The average yoga practitioner spends about $90 per month on yoga and practices yoga at least 2-3 times per week. Furthermore, 37% of yoga enthusiasts practice yoga with their children as well.

Yoga is becoming more popular as people realize its immense benefits and make it a priority to practice regularly.

However, there continue to be many myths about yoga that are untrue for newcomers. Here are some myths that you probably heard about yoga.

Yoga is All About Religion

There are some people who believe yoga is only suitable for those who have religious ties. Yoga does share many practices and goals with Buddhism, Hinduism, and Jainism, but it's actually closer to science than religion, since it connects everyone under the banner of wellbeing.

Therefore, yoga is free from any and all forms of discrimination, including ones based on ethnicity, racial bias, or gender. It integrates the mind, body, and spirit and offers the opportunity for wellbeing and integration, regardless of age.

You Need to be Flexible

Yoga is typically marketed as only for flexible people. There is no truth to this statement. Social media feeds to the world the stereotypical image of tough poses being done by youthful people and others who look very athletic. However, this isn't the complete story of yoga.

There is no reason for anyone not to practice yoga, but especially those who are considered inflexible. As part of the yoga practice, you'll achieve flexibility in your mind and body. It's also possible to practice a variety of yoga while being seated in a chair.

Yoga isn't Even a Workout

People often make this mistake when they know little about a subject or are simply too hasty and make a quick judgment. In fact, yoga can be an intense workout that can leave you covered in sweat! It can be very challenging. Yoga can also help tone muscles, strengthen, and even burn calories. An all-around workout that focuses on the body and the mind.

People with Asthma Can't Do It

Asthma sufferers may not be capable of doing all forms of yoga. However, yoga is still effective for those who have asthma, specifically chair yoga.

Yoga poses can provide health benefits for individuals having a hard time with breathing, and help them gain incredible physical and mental strength from practicing the art. In reality, yoga practice is beneficial to those who actually do it.

All You Do is Pose

There is no denying that yoga poses look incredible, but the true practice of yoga is about elevating your consciousness at a much deeper level. Mind, body, and emotions are united by yoga. A positive attitude helps you achieve your goals, reduces stress, and makes you more happy in life. A relaxing massage will help you unwind and will allow you to find peace and tranquility inside. Meditation and breathing exercises are also part of yoga, even though it's mainly a physical practice.

Only Young Folks Do Yoga

No particular age group is excluded from yoga. A number of yoga classes are offered for seniors that are designed specifically to focus on their health and well-being. People are likely to develop this misconception when only considering what the media pushes in society. Everyone can practice yoga, regardless of age. This book is a prime example of the types of yoga available for older adults.

There are many examples where older practitioners of yoga, who started their journey in their 60s, have reached the point where they can perform complicated poses with relative ease and perfection. Practice makes perfect, and yoga is not different in that aspect. A person can begin practicing yoga at any age.

It's Just For Girls

Another misconception about yoga is the idea that it's only beneficial to women. Men have debunked the claim that yoga is primarily practiced by women. There are approximately 25% to 35% of yoga practitioners in the US who are men, and their numbers are only increasing every year. Yoga classes for men are also taught by yogis and yoga experts.

Yoga became popular in Western societies around the 1980s when it became a worldwide phenomenon. Nevertheless, as more and more people gained widespread awareness and popularity for the practice, myths and misconceptions also grew, naturally.

The myths listed above about yoga are not true at all. It would be our pleasure if you could see yoga as a complete system for all humanity without distinctions based on race, class, gender, and age.

Benefits of Daily Chair Yoga

Eases neck tension
Improves balance
Improves mental clarity
Promotes relaxation

Low impact on joints
Improves flexibility
Promotes weight loss
Relieves inflammation
Promotes ankle and foot mobility
Increases knee mobility and range
Boost shoulder joint movement
Strengthen arms
Reduces symptoms of anxiety
Builds stamina and strengthen muscles
Lowers risk of falling

According to the Center for Disease Control and Prevention, the leading cause of injury and death for older adults of 65+ years is falling. The rate of death among people 75+ has increased from 2014 to 2016, according to a study published in the Journal of the American Medical Association. Another alarming reality is the amount of medications older adults are consuming. Over the years, these increased doses tend to result in lightheadedness, muscle reduction, and losing balance, in many situations. Yoga has become an important topic among doctors that recommend yoga. At Manhattan Physical Medicine and Rehabilitation in New York City, Loren Fisher, MD, regularly prescribes yoga as part of the patient's medicinal treatment. Side effects of traditional western medicines can be offset by chair yoga.

Even the fear of falling has grief-stricken many older adults and loved ones. The debilitating feeling that your next step one morning may be fatal is enough to cause procrastination. You may find yourself avoiding activities you long to do from the fear of losing your balance. Almost half older adults have reported their fear of falling and the concern that lead them to miss out on warm memories with their family (Podewitz, J. 2019).

All the more reason routine chair yoga can alleviate the worry that plagues your movement. Let's begin the journey to a new, refreshing lifestyle that will grant you more freedom than you could've imagined possible.

Welcome to chair yoga.

MAKE THE MOST OUT OF CHAIR YOGA

So now that you have made the decision to change your daily habits for the better, it's imperative that you make the most from this decision. The level of commitment will make a difference in your results. My grandmother always told me "Procrastinate today, feel it tomorrow". While I never listened to those words growing up as a child, I also never failed to feel the terrible result from my procrastination. As an adult, I pass on the same message to other adults. The message is easier to swallow with love, care, and guidance.

Let's get started!

How To Prepare

For starters, we need a chair (of course). Not just any old chair. It is vital for the beginner to have a chair without a cushion. That's right. I know you are tempted to get as comfortable as possible with the memory foam seat. And while that may seem ideal, that is not ideal for chair yoga. Your position is key in these poses, and a cushioned seat may alter your pose. Make sure the chair is straight back, as well. Avoid the La-Z Boy chair. If applicable, a wheelchair will do splendidly. Use a chair without arms because you will be less restricted in the poses.

It's recommended that you reserve a place in your home for your routine. This doesn't have to be a separate room strictly for yoga. It should, however, have distance from any distractions nearby. Distractions such as TVs and electronic-anything, really. The ideal location is a placid, soothing "happy place" in your home.

While this may sound like hippy talk, a truly healthy environment is relaxing on your mind and inevitably your body. You don't need to be a flower child to know that the most relaxing place on earth tends to be nature-esque. Chair yoga on a beach may not be an option, but a quiet room, less distractions, or an area away from hallways and loud noises will make a world of difference.

Make sure there is a mirror in front of you, for beginning purposes. You won't always have to look at yourself throughout this journey. Right now, you are new to these poses. You need to check in with your positioning.

Clothes

You should wear nothing that will restrict your movement. If you are wearing clothes that are too heavy, that's already a problem. Strive for comfort. Go barefoot if you must. There is such a connection between your bare feet and the ground beneath you. As we wear shoes constantly throughout the day, we are disconnected from the earth beneath us. A large focus of your chair yoga will center around being grounded. There is a difference between wearing shoes, socks, and bare feet touching the ground. It's why we prefer our feet bare against the floors of our homes (unless you're cold or the floors need some cleaning). We reach a new level of relaxation when there is nothing restricting our feet from touching the ground. This level of groundedness will be your ally for yoga. You will feel the difference.

If you must wear shoes, do so with rubber sole shoes. Avoid socks, especially on hardwood floors. That is a recipe for slips and falls. If you are executing your poses on a rug or carpet, the socks are less of a danger.

Essentially Comfortable

It's recommended that these routines be done in the morning, but is that always possible? Making this a morning habit may be great for one person, but not ideal for the next. Chair yoga is all about your personal preference when it comes to being comfortable. If you are more active at night, then this will be your moment in the evening. If you can commit to a morning schedule, then do so. Your body isn't the same as the next one. Know your body. Know your comforts. Know your limitations. The time of day you choose will be yours to make a habit. You must have consistency, or these routines will never have their full effect on your body. It's unfair to ask for change of yourself if you are not willing to put in the work for change.

What about some extra comforts? What about listening to music, as we mentioned earlier? Here's the thing. Some folks are more comfortable with a delicate melody in the background for their yoga. For some, music clears the mind. It brings tranquility, and that is a beautiful way to begin the day or end the night. I will never be against music during yoga! However, be careful to choose a playlist that isn't distracting you in all the wrong ways. These routines should calm you, not bring about memories that bring anger or frustration. Think of this as background music. It isn't the focus. If the music contains lyrics, be careful to not let the lyrics distract you. I recommend music and yoga in your routine.

Pairing Yoga with Music

As a species, we are inextricably linked to music. Music pervades all cultures, regardless of their level of development. History has proven it true, and it has been true throughout a lifetime. It doesn't matter how talented or how off-key we are, we sing, we hum, we sway, we dance, we bounce.

Music can be distinguished from noise by the brain, and the nervous system can react to rhythm, repetition, tones and tunes. Does this biological accident serve a purpose or is it a biological accident? We can't know for sure. Music is still suggested to be good for human health and performance by a variety of studies.

Music might also improve cardiovascular health by reducing stress hormones, lowering blood pressure, and slowing down heart rate. Adding music in the background of your yoga practice may have the ability to make your practice a bit more encouraging if your motivation relates to improving your physical health, or your mental health.

Imagine how beneficial chair yoga music is if simply listening to music while not exercising already offers an abundance of health benefits.

INTRODUCTION TO FRIENDLY EXERCISES

"Chair Yoga has a unique way of isolating the area around the joints and core to gently work them to build strength and flexibility" - *Julie Smith*

The beginner must start with the most attainable routines initially. The best beginning is the warm up stages. These stages focus on breathing. With your comfortable chair ready, your quiet setting prepared, and musical choice (if any) started, you are ready to practice deep breaths. In order to make your breathing more even, try counting to three or four as you inhale through your nose, and then again as you exhale from your mouth.

FRIENDLY POSES

Seated Mountain Pose
Cat Cow Position
Seated Row
Knee Extensions
Seated March
Toe Lifts
Overhead Press
Raised Hands
Warrior One Clap
Slight Spinal Twist

Seated Mountain Pose

IMPROVES SPINAL FLEXIBILITY

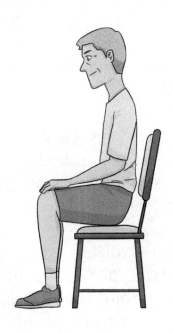

Instructions

1. The starter position. You will be sitting up tall while you take your breaths.

2. With every exhale, take a quick mental note of where your tension lives. Release any hold you have (shoulders, elbows, fingers, etc.). Feel free to give your toes a wiggle. Any point of your body that is holding onto your stress, this is the time to check in. Release the tension. Inhale. Count. Exhale. Count.

3. Make sure your hands are on your thighs. Feel your whole body on the chair. Keep your knees above your ankles with little room between your knees.

4. As you exhale again, roll your shoulders down your back, pulling your belly button in toward your spine. Keep your arms relaxed. Your hands should be relaxed on your thighs.

5. Your feet are the roots, your legs the bark. You are sitting tall. This is the mountain pose.

Cat Cow Position

IMPROVES POSTURE AND BALANCE

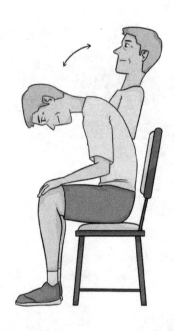

Instructions

1.Take deep, even breaths. Sit so your spine is long, feet still planted.

2.As you inhale, arch your back and allow the shoulders to gently drop down your back, bringing your shoulder blades to your back. This is the cow position.

3.On your exhale, round your spine and drop your chin to your chest, which will let your shoulder and head come forward. This is the cat position.

Seated Row

*IMPROVES POSTURE AND
RELAXES SHOULDERS*

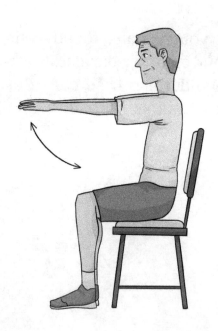

Instructions

1.Hold your arms out straight in front of you. Keep them at shoulder level with your thumbs pointed towards the ceiling.

2.Bring your elbows back and squeeze the shoulder blades together until your upper arms align with the sides of your torso.

3.Extend your arms back to starter position. Repeat the set three times.

Knee Extensions

*RELIEVES CHRONIC KNEE PAIN
AND HYPEREXTENSION*

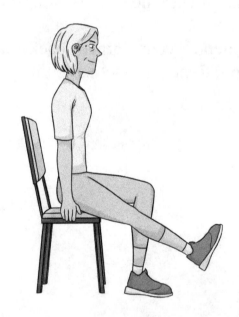

Instructions

1.Both knees kept together with your feet on the floor, straighten one leg out in front of you.

2.Hold for one second, then gently bend the leg back to rest on the floor.

3.Repeat steps with the next leg. Repeat the set three times.

Seated March

*STRENGTHENS CORE AND
PELVIC MUSCLES*

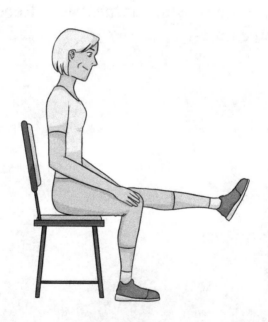

Instructions

1.Lift one leg, knee bent to your comfort zone.

2.Put the foot down slowly.

3.Repeat with the next leg. Repeat the set three times.

Toe Lifts

IMPROVES FOOT ALIGNMENT

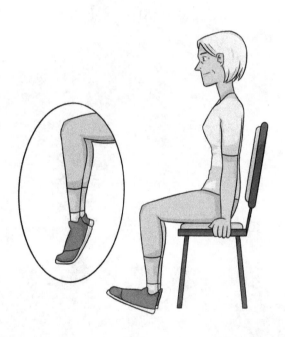

Instructions

1.Lift your toes, both feet, while keeping your heels on the floor.

2.Then, put your toes down and lift your heels, carefully applying a small squeeze to your calf muscles as you do this.

3.Put your heels down. Repeat this set three times.

Overhead Press

*STRENGTHENS LOWER BACK
AND ABS*

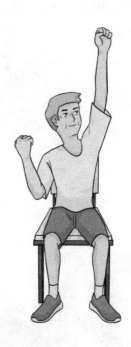

Instructions

1.Bend your arms upwards so your wrists are next to your shoulders.

2.With careful control, air punch diagonally up and across your body with the first arm. Slightly rotate your torso in the same direction as you air punch.

3.Bend your arm back and bring it in after the air punch, then do so with the next arm.

4.Repeat the set three times.

Raised Hands

IMPROVES STABILITY

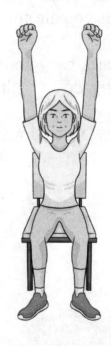

Instructions

1.Raise your arms straight up towards the ceiling. Maintain your upper body posture with the shoulders relaxed.

2.Keep your rib cage sitting naturally over the hips. Count to three before lowering your arms again.

3.Repeat the set three times.

Warrior One Clap

IMPROVES CIRCULATION,
STRENGTHENS SHOULDERS, ARMS,
LEGS, ABDOMEN

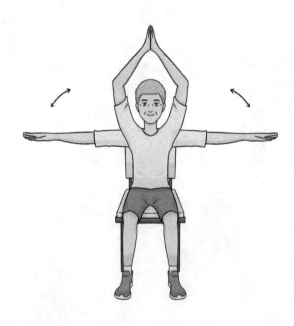

Instructions

1.Lift your arms out to the sides, then raise your hands above your head and have your hands meet.

2.Intertwine your fingers together, keeping your fingers pointed and thumbs out. You should be pointing directly at the ceiling.

3.Roll your shoulders away from your ears. Take a few deep breaths here before returning your arms gently back to your sides.

4.Repeat this set three times.

Slight Spinal Twist

IMPROVES BACK FLEXIBILITY

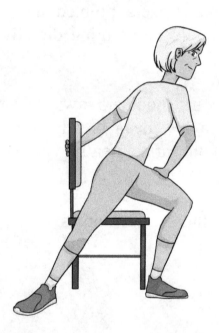

Instructions

1.Shift sideways on the chair, facing left.

2.Twist your torso gently towards the left, the amount that is possible only.

3.Hold onto the back of the chair.

4.Lengthen spine on each inhale and twist, exhale for five breaths.

5.Move your legs around to the right, repeat.

Tips

Always inhale before every movement, then exhale on the next. You should fall into a pattern of inhaling to execute, exhaling to release. This is extremely important.

Your body will want to tense up with every motion you make. In order to alleviate the stress building in your muscles, the deep breathes must be made throughout the motions. This may seem tedious at first, but when it becomes a habit, you will focus more on the flow between one pose into the next without thinking of the breaths very often. This, however, won't be the case until you have made inhaling/exhaling on every motion your second nature.

The first few routines won't be entirely smooth, and that is perfectly fine. These are beginner motions. We start out with 3 set repetitions per exercise, however, these can be adjusted. You may increase/decrease the sets to your comfortability. Never push yourself beyond limitations.

In the beginning, you either believe that you can do anything because it may not seem so difficult, or you may doubt your abilities to ever progress and advance. You will find that it's easier to be patient with yourself when you work through the beginning stages. Practice and discipline are required to master difficult poses, and they don't happen overnight. Understanding that everyone is unique also means being patient when it comes to particular poses you may never be able to master.

Beginners may have difficulty keeping up with the movements of each pose, and may even worry about falling over. By becoming more proficient, you will realize how vital it is to breathe correctly in every aspect of your practice and every action you take. Paying attention to your breath allows you to balance your body and stay focused. Several breathing techniques are available for you to practice as you become more skilled in order to find expansion in your inhalations and stability in your exhalations. There will be further details on deep breathing later.

Increasing your practice to the intermediate level benefits both your body and your mind. You can progress in your yoga practice and improve your focus and concentration by practicing meditation, which will be discussed further in upcoming chapters. It will also make you feel more calm in the chair.

BEGINNER POSITIONS

"Anybody can breathe therefore anybody can practice yoga." - T.K.V Desikachar

Whenever you start regular home practices, you should pay attention to your body's signals. What feels good one day could be excruciating the next, as chronic pain conditions can change from day to day. Any pose that causes sharp, stabbing pain should be modified or changed by using an appropriate prop.

Take your time exploring the ones below. You may find yourself feeling discouraged if some of the poses are too challenging for you when you're just starting an exercise routine. As you practice, slow down, breathe, and remember that these

movements will gradually become easier and
more comfortable.

BEGINNER POSES

Half-Moon Rolls

Hand-to-Head Rolls

Deep Twist

Half Sun Salutation

Rag Doll

Core Builder

Single Leg Forward Bend

Pigeon Pose

Goddess Pose

Shoulder Release

Half-Moon Rolls

PROMOTES FLEXIBILITY

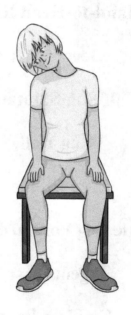

Instructions

1.Keeping your spinal cord straight, hands on thighs, calm breaths, gently drop your neck to the side, ear to shoulder.

2.Move your head further down across your chest, your next ear to your next shoulder.

3.Create half moons with this rotation.

Hand-to-Head Rolls

NECK STRENGTHENING

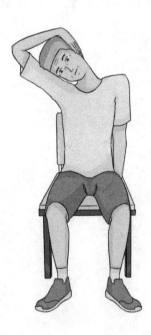

Instructions

1.Lower your left ear to your left shoulder.

2.Raise your left hand and gently place it down on your right ear. Straighten your right arm, slightly raising it away from your body in a straight line.

3.Take three deep breaths here.

4.Release and repeat on the next side.

Deep Twist

*IMPROVES BACK MUSCLE
FLEXIBILITY*

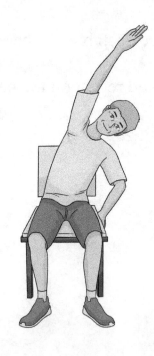

Instructions

1.Move your right hand to the outer edge of the chair, crossing your body to the right, grip the chair.

2.Reach your left arm up to the sky.

3.Move into a side bend. Take three deep even breaths.

4.Come back up, bring your left hand to the back of the chair and twist your body to the left. Reach your right arm to the sky.

5.Keep that stretch for three deep breaths. Be sure not to slouch in this exercise.

Half Sun Salutation

STRENGTHEN BACK MUSCLES

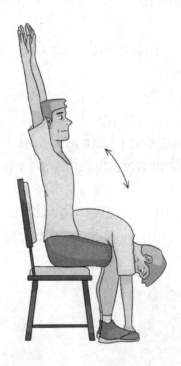

Instructions

1.Raise your hands out and reach up to the sky.

2.As your arms fall, drop your upper half body lower as well, head towards the knees (to the amount you can).

3.Relax head, neck. Raise your head and back halfway up only. Pause a moment, then drop back down.

4.Raise again, hold, drop gently again.

5.Release position.

Rag Doll

SPINAL STRETCH

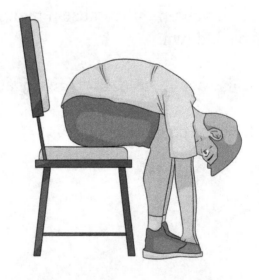

Instructions

1.Turn the whole body to the left, legs straight out.

2.Gently drop your upper body, head towards knees.

3.Let your arms stretch out straight, past your knees. Stretch as much as you can.

4.Use your hands to aid in coming back up.

Core Builder

STRENGTHENS THE HIP AND CORE

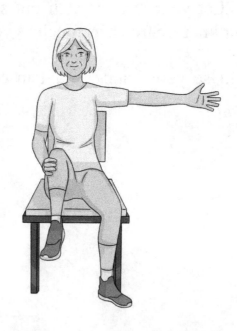

Instructions

1.Facing forward, raise your knee up, hold your front shin with your hands. Hold it there and rotate your ankle.

2.After a few rotations in both directions, let go of your shin with your left hand.

3.Stretch your left arm away from your body. Return your left hand to your shin, and release your right arm, stretch away from your body for a few breaths.

4.Then release both of your hands from your shin, keeping the knee up without support.

5.Breathe evenly once, then return your hands to your shin and lower your leg.

6.Repeat for the next leg.

Single Leg Forward Bend

IMPROVES RANGE OF HAMSTRING MOTION

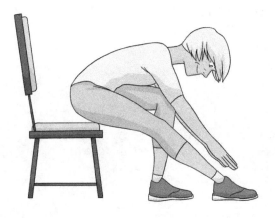

Instructions

1.Sit at the front edge of the seat with your left foot flat on the floor.

2.Extend the right leg out in front of you, lengthen your body, drawing the lower belly towards your spine. Fold forward over your stretched leg.

3.Breathe evenly three times and inhale coming back to the upright position.

4.Repeat on the other side.

Pigeon Pose

IMPROVES GLUTE FLEXIBILITY

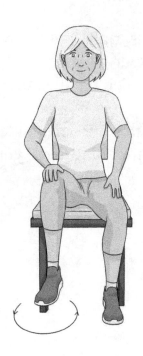

Instructions

1.Lift your right foot a few inches off the floor, take hold of your right knee and make circles in both directions.

2.Repeat with your left foot.

3.Cross your right ankle over your left shin and use your hand to hold the position. Hold for three even breaths, then release.

4.Repeat with your left ankle. If you can cross your entire ankle over your knee, feel free to do so.

Goddess Pose

OPENS HIPS/MIDSECTION

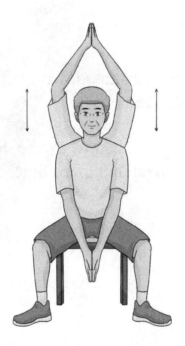

Instructions

1.Open your legs as wide as possible, heels in and toes pointed out. Hips and knees open.

2.Raise your hands to the air outwards, arms stretched to the ceiling and palm together.

3.Bring your hands down in front of you, still palmed together.

4.Return your hands to the top of your thighs and repeat one more time.

Shoulder Release

*IMPROVES UPPER BODY
FLEXIBILITY*

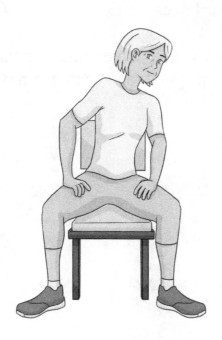

Instructions

1.With open legs, heels in, toes out, keep your hands on your knees and drop your right shoulder down, and slightly turn your upper body left.

2.Use your right hand to add a small push against your knees for extra stretch.

3.Breathe evenly five times, then return your body upright and execute the next side.

Tips

Yoga is not for people who can perform each pose without effort. You should be content with where you are right now, but you should also continue to grow, evolve, and push your limits. Yoga tends to require the same poses and the same teachers, which is why it can be easy to become complacent. Despite that, you may be worried about taking the step from beginning to intermediate yoga.

Consistency is key. In order to move up from beginner's yoga to intermediate level, you must be consistently in that chair. When you're getting used to your new routine, your yoga practice is likely to be sporadic at first. In the beginning, you're probably more likely to practice more often, since you're much more eager to practice. However, a few weeks later, you will find it difficult to get back to the chair. Back to the quiet, peaceful setting you created when you began to build this habit. Life takes many turns, and we sometimes simply lose steam. To become an intermediate practitioner, you must practice consistently. You must try to stick to your routine. If you find your morning schedule no longer works, it may be time to change it. If the evenings have become more relaxed, then switch to evenings instead. The moment your routine returns habitually, you will progress to the next level.

In intermediate yoga, it's essential to have a strong core. Beginners and intermediates differ in regard to achieving a better solid core. There are layers of muscles that protect your abdominals in addition to the central muscles in your body. If you have a solid core, you will be able to achieve advanced yoga postures.

ADVANCED POSITIONS

"You are only as young as your spine is flexible." - Joseph Pilates

When you are ready to enter the more advanced positions of chair yoga, your breathing with every movement should be second nature. This isn't a race. Approach this stage with certainty and confidence. If you have tiredness, heat sensitivity, poor balance, a serious lung, heart, or bone condition, avoid aggressive yoga techniques and difficult poses. If you have serious spine issues, such as a herniated disc, or if you have undergone muscle surgery, consult your doctor further before moving into advanced chair yoga. These positions will always be available when you are prepared.

ADVANCED POSES

Side Angle Pose
Warrior I
Warrior II
Reverse Warrior
Hero's Pose
Lunge Pose
Half-Splits
Triangle Pose
Down Dog
Savasana/Final Relaxation

Side Angle Pose

FLEXIBILITY FOR LIMITED MOBILITY

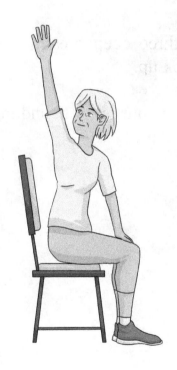

Instructions

1.Bring your hands to your floor, or block, or to your knees.

2.While inhaling, extend your right arm to the sky, while your left hand stays on the ground.

3.Take three deep breaths and turn your neck to look up.

4.Reverse your left arm and inhale back to the forward fold.

Warrior I

POWER AND STABILITY

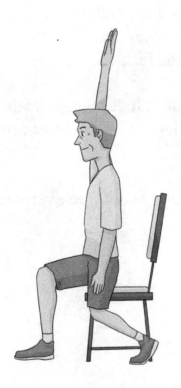

Instructions

1.While swinging your left leg behind you, keep your right leg over the side of the chair.

2.Put the sole of your left foot on the floor parallel to the seat of the chair, then straighten the left leg.

3.As you inhale, keep your torso over your right leg and raise your arms up to the ceiling.

4.Pause and take three even breaths.

Warrior II

POWER AND STABILITY

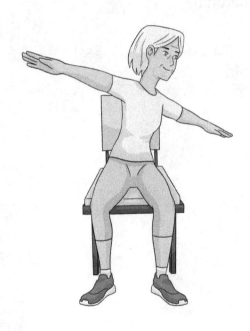

Instructions

1.As you exhale, bring your right arm forward and your left arm back.

2.As you turn your torso left, draw your left hip back and align your left hip with the front of the chair.

3.Focus on your right fingertips for a three second hold.

Reverse Warrior

STRENGTHENS MID-SECTION

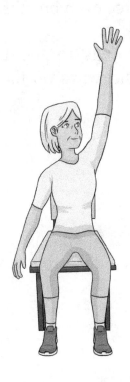

Instructions

1.Have your left arm come down your left leg and lift your right arm up to the ceiling on an inhale.

2.Hold for three even breaths.

3.Bring both legs to the front of your chair, then sit sideways on the chair facing left.

Hero's Pose

TARGETS LARGE QUADS

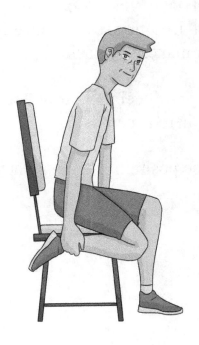

Instructions

1.Shift to the edge of your chair so that your right leg is off the chair. Hold the edge of the chair with your left hand for balance.

2.Lean to the left as you bend your right knee, then take your foot with your right hand. Feel free to use a strap around your foot if that makes this easier.

3.Bring your heel to your buttock. Release slightly if there is pain.

4.Release position and do the next leg.

Lunge Pose

KNEE PROBLEMS

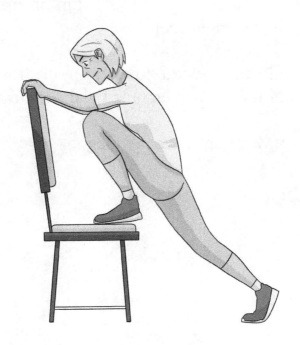

Instructions

1. Stand in front of the chair, arm's length away.

2. Turn the chair 90 degrees and hold back if balancing is a problem. Bring your weight onto your left foot and step up on the chair with your right foot.

3. Lean forward towards your front leg. Hold for a few even breaths, then release.

4. Move on to the next leg.

Half-Splits

BALANCE

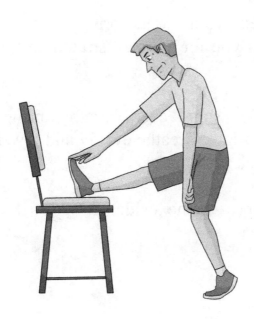

Instructions

1.From lunge pose, straighten your front leg and rest your heel on the chair.

2.Remain in this position to work on balance.

3.Flex your foot, bringing your toes towards you for an extra stretch on the back legs.

4.After some even breaths, bring your torso upright. Breathe evenly and lower your foot back to the floor.

5.Repeat the next side.

Triangle Pose

SIDE STRETCHES

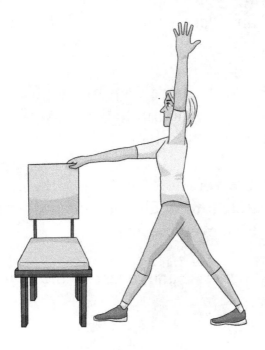

Instructions

1. Standing next to your chair with the right side of your body closest to the chair, have your feet three to four feet apart.

2. Turn your right foot with your toes to the chair. Plant your left foot at a 45 degree angle.

3. Raise your arms up to shoulder height. Reach your right arm to the back of the chair or the seat of the chair.

4. Have your left hand reach the ceiling as you stretch through the left side of your body. Five even breaths here.

5. Slowly rise and repeat on the next side.

Down Dog

BACK STRETCH

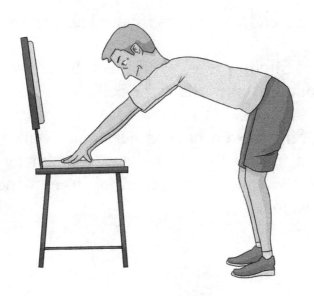

Instructions

1.Facing the chair, lift your arms over your head.

2.Exhale while you bend forward and put the palms of your hands on the seat of the chair.

3.Bend your knees if your legs are tight.

4.Slightly walk your feet back and lift your hips upwards to the ceiling.

5.Five even breaths here, then walk your feet toward the chair, bend your knees and gently roll your spine up to a standing position.

Savasana/Final Relaxation

TRANSITIONING TO YOUR DAY OR EVENING

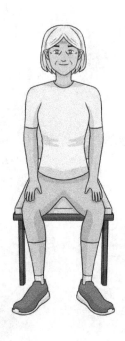

Instructions

1.Towards the end of your practice, sit with your eyes closed and hands in your lap.

2.Savasana helps your body absorb all the benefits you have gained from the poses you have done throughout the day or night. It helps you to transition into the remainder of your day or helps you sleep at night. A much needed last pose, especially in advance stages.

MEDITATION

It's impossible to venture into chair yoga, or yoga at all, without mentioning meditation.

Meditation has been used to help individuals feel more at ease since ancient times. Meditation has grown in popularity in recent years as a result of its scientifically established advantages. It is a technique for teaching your mind to concentrate, relax, and redirect your thoughts.

For seniors, meditation keeps their brains calm and active, allowing them to age gracefully. Meditation can provide these unexpected health advantages by infusing awareness into a senior's mind, body, and soul. It lowers and regulates blood pressure, improves immune system function to regulate cortisol levels, reduces the risk of stress-related illnesses such as diabetes, hypertension, and high cholesterol by reducing muscular tension and pains that are commonly connected with feeling worried or nervous.

Through yoga's meditation, here is an in depth look at the benefits.

Stress and Anxiety Reducer

One of the best-known benefits of yoga's meditation is its ability to reduce stress and anxiety. Studies conducted in 2016 report that 21.6% of people used meditation for stress relief, and 29.2% for anxiety relief (Senior Lifestyle, 2020).

Meditating can help you eliminate inner thoughts that can exert strain on your emotional well-being. You can manage stress symptoms throughout the day if you maintain a good sense of self-awareness and tranquility.

Contain the Pain

According to studies, 11% of the adult population in the United States suffers from chronic pain each year (Senior Lifestyle,

2020). Because our physical experience of pain is related to our brains, it might be amplified when we're stressed. Because mindfulness meditation helps you to focus on breathing and how your body feels in the present moment, it's a fantastic approach to manage discomfort. Your body becomes aligned with neural system rhythms when you breathe up to six times each minute. With these 30 chair yoga movements, you may also learn how to treat joint discomfort.

Memory Loss

Meditation has been shown to reduce symptoms of memory loss. It has been shown to boost telomerase, an enzyme essential to slow the progression of illnesses like Alzheimer's, by 43%. Furthermore, studies discovered that those who meditate on a daily basis may tap into the strength or emotion of their subconscious mind, allowing their brain to retain more knowledge (Senior Lifestyle, 2020).

Improvement of Attention Span

These techniques that are focused can improve the strength and durability of your attention span. Meditation has the ability to prevent age related mental impairments, according to a 2017 research study published in the Journal of Cognitive Enhancement. The participants of this study were put through a variety of meditation training exercises, including maintaining object concentration, mindful breathing methods, and creating pleasant feelings for others and for oneself. The study's findings revealed that the training improved the participants' emotional well-being and helped them perform better on activities requiring focus and attention.

The goal of each meditation practice is to alter one's state of mind and channel normal waking consciousness in a more positive direction. Turning inwards and focusing on the inner self is what meditation entails. Mental health issues should never be a concern for you if you meditate frequently, and both your mental and physical self will improve.

It has been demonstrated that meditation, via deliberation and contemplation, is one of the safest complementary and alternative medical practices. Meditation isn't only about replacing the bad ideas with the positive thoughts. Instead, it provides a welcome break from the usual diatribe. The state of physical and mental well-being is what we refer to as mental health. It's nothing more than a description of any taught socially adaptable behavior that enables people to function well in life. Meditation is a great method for achieving a state of psychological well-being, one's true potential, and the capacity to maintain rewarding, meaningful relationships.

One of the most significant advantages of meditation is the reduction of tension. Regular meditation will help you achieve a higher degree of relaxation and introspection. The benefits of meditation may help you live a life that is quiet, serene, joyful, and relaxed if you wish to be free of continual worry, pressure, and stress.

Even 10 minutes every day might help you relax. Now we can conclude that if you practice meditation on a regular basis, you will be able to concentrate better.

At the end of your session, you can finish the practice by resting your joined hands in front of your belly or on your lap. Clasp your hands together and stretch the fingers, pushing them together and pointing them forward. Take deep, slow breaths here. Breathe in through the nose, out through the mouth. This works because you are drawing the breath's energy downward and lengthening the exhale, which is both grounding and soothing.

DEEP BREATHING

As mentioned earlier, breathing carries your energy. You will execute every movement in yoga by inhaling and exhaling. Knowing how to conduct deep breaths will help you move in and out of every pose.

Complete Exhalation

Exhale as you sit up straight. Take a deep breath and relax your abdominal muscles. Your lungs fill with breath. Feel your belly expand. Continue inhaling until you feel your chest expand as you take a deep breath. Hold your breath for a second before gently exhaling, pushing your belly button in to feel the final breath leave your lungs. For five minutes, close your eyes, relax, and focus solely on your breathing.

Breathing While Humming

Follow the directions for Complete Exhalation, but when it comes time to exhale, hum as you let go of the air. As you hum the last of the air out of your body, pull your abdominal muscles in. Relax for two to three minutes while performing this breathing exercise.

Tai Chi Chuan Breathing

This breathing exercise is based on Tai Chi Chuan, a Chinese martial art. Take three quick breaths in, lifting your arms shoulder height in front of you on the first, shoulder height at your sides on the second, and above your head on the third. After that, slowly exhale and return your arms to your sides. Aim for 10-12 reps. Stop doing the exercise if you feel dizzy.

Breathing via the Diaphragm

The most convenient position to do this breathing exercise is on your back. Place one hand on your stomach above your navel and the other above it. Now focus on breathing deeply from your diaphragm. You are completing this exercise correctly if you can see the hand over your navel rising before the hand above it. For five minutes, relax and focus on your breathing.

Breathing of the Feet

This is a breathing routine as well as an active relaxing method. As your chest and diaphragm rise and fall in unison, focus on your breathing. Allow yourself to calm your mind by breathing normally. Imagine your stress and anxiety flowing down your body and out via your feet as you breathe. Repeat till you've reached a state of relaxation.

Breathing of Buteyko

This practice, named after Russian physiologist Konstantin Buteyko, is very beneficial for those who suffer from respiratory issues such as asthma. Begin by finding a comfortable resting posture in a quiet area and concentrating on taking shallow breaths gently through your nose instead of deep breaths. This approach can help those who are having an asthma attack or are in a stressful environment slow down the cycle of fast gasping breaths.

YOUR HEALTH MATTERS

As you venture through this journey of chair yoga, it will be natural to gain insight on your mental health. This is a very necessary step when practicing yoga.

How long has it been since you deeply considered your mental health? Do you have any doubts? As a senior, you may not think about mental health as often as you used to. In reality, many people lack knowledge about the best approach to starting a discussion about it. Surely, you aren't the only one who doesn't put this topic high on your list of concerns. However, it might be worth it. Perhaps you will gain new insights into life through exploring this topic.

It is imperative that you maintain your health. It can be influenced by mental factors as well, so why ignore them? It's no secret that each of us has an inner life filled with strong beliefs, ever-changing perceptions, unique emotions, and precious beliefs. These things determine how we act and how we define ourselves as human beings. Our mental health, relationships, and overall quality of life can also be affected by them.

Therefore, if you pay attention to your mental health, you are more likely to make positive changes. Mental health plays a major role in our lives, regardless of our age. You will be able to thrive more if you understand it.

Start the Conversation

Would you ignore a broken arm and continue your day as if nothing happened? Probably not. If the pain became too intense, it would be unbearable. The problem would only get worse if left unattended. Therefore, it should be treated. You'd probably do everything in your power to prevent it from happening again. Everything seems pretty straightforward, doesn't it?

How about if it was a more hidden injury? How would you feel if it was your mind? Is there any way you could recognize something is wrong? What would you do even if you realized that you had a problem? Would you seek help right away, or would you ignore it as much as possible until it got worse? The answer to those questions is probably not as straightforward as one might think. Mental health is a subject many people dodge and downplay.

Many seniors and the elderly are misunderstood or marginalized due to mental health issues. This is regrettable. You need to be at least as healthy mentally as you are physically. Untreated mental health problems and mental disorders may make it difficult to lead a fulfilling and enjoyable life, develop meaningful relationships, or achieve your daily goals. Symptoms can also make it more difficult to recover from wounds or treat pre-existing illnesses.

Achieving and maintaining a better quality of life begins by taking your mental well-being seriously.

Common Mental Health Conditions in Seniors

About 15% of all adults over the age of 60 experience some type of mental illness, according to the World Health Organization (WHO). There is always someone who has experienced conditions like those below - even if they have kept it in private. There is no reason to consider any of these issues normal with aging. It's neither a cause for shame, nor a reason to hide them. Seeking help, even starting with chair yoga, can often help treat and manage these conditions. Elderly and senior adults commonly suffer from mental health problems, such as:

Depression

Geriatric mental health issues are important because older adults have a heightened risk of depression. It's normal to feel sad sometimes. The problem with depression goes far beyond that. Depression is most commonly characterized by a persistently low mood, which may not always appear as madness. Other ongoing feelings they might experience are anxiety, guilt, anger, shame, emptiness, worthlessness, irritability, and hopelessness. Their previously favorite activities no longer bring them joy. Suicide may also be a result of feeling dull and apathetic about life. Age is an important factor in suicide rates among elderly men (Harvard, 2021).

Anxiety disorders

We all experience temporary worries and fears. Others have persistent feelings of anxiety that are triggered by certain sorts of situations or that never go away. This makes them incapable of performing normal everyday activities. The symptoms they experience can also get worse with time and cause more interference in their lives. Anxiety disorders come in many forms. Seniors are generally more prone to anxiety disorders, including generalized anxiety disorder, social anxiety disorder, panic disorder, and obsessive-compulsive disorder. Anxiety disorders are often associated with depression.

Dementia

There are several types of dementia besides Alzheimer's disease, which is important for people to know. The symptoms of dementia can include memory loss and behavioral changes, as well as confusion, personality changes, and difficulty communicating. Rather than classifying dementia as a mental illness, some professionals prefer to classify it as a brain disorder. Regardless, the impact of it on a person's mental well-being is considerable no matter how it's being classified. Because of this, mental disorders like dementia should be among the topics we consider when discussing elderly health - even if they're difficult to describe and discuss.

It's worth noting that depression may resemble dementia, but they are vastly different. However, the distinctions between these two situations might be difficult to spot. People with dementia lose their mental sharpness, but it may also happen to people who are depressed. The key differences: Slow mental deterioration, confusion, markedly decreased motor abilities, and problems with short-term memory are all signs of dementia. Depression, on the other hand, might lead to a faster (but more restricted) mental deterioration, showing as issues with attention and energy. People suffering from depression may also be aware that they're having memory problems. People with dementia, on the other hand, are frequently ignorant of their memory difficulties.

Yoga as Treatment for Depression, Anxiety, and Dementia

As we age, we accumulate loss. Throughout our lives we experience the loss of loved ones. Our parents, friends, spouses. Our health and movement also change throughout the years. During our sleep, we may experience anxiety or depression, and worry about the next moment ahead.

As mentioned earlier, yoga isn't just good for the body, but it can help reduce anxiety and depression.

During a six month yoga course, adults reported positive changes in mood, fatigue, and other quality-of-life indicators, according to a 2006 study published in Alternative Therapies in Health and Medicine.

Yoga was also found to help adults with depression develop coping strategies and regain a sense of connectedness, according to research published in 2013 in the Archives of Psychiatric Nursing. During the research study, Patricia Anne Kinser and her colleagues found that yoga offered additional benefits in lowering ruminations, in addition to reducing depression for all 27 participants.

In a recent report from Florida Atlantic University study, chair yoga can assist in the improvement of quality of life with dementia patients. The study consisted of older adults with moderate-to-severe dementia. For 12 weeks, the participants attended a 45 minute session. They attended two times a week. The results revealed that more than 97% of the participants were fully engaged in each session. The study lead, Juyoung Park, Ph.D. expressed his fascination. The participants, prior to the session, were agitated but their demeanor completely changed when the instructor began to demonstrate the yoga poses. They did not understand the verbal instructions due to their cognitive impairment that is paired with advanced dementia, they did, however, follow the instructor's poses.

Understanding the Risk Factors

Mental health disorders can be caused by a variety of factors. In reality, they're rarely triggered by a single factor. Many factors - social, physical, and psychological - can interact to cause a mental illness that disrupts one's life. Someone's current state of being doesn't dictate the future. You, or someone you care about may develop mental health problems in the future. Be cautious of these risk factors:

Medical problems

There are many medical conditions that can lend a hand to the development of mental health concerns, which includes depression. There are other examples like arthritis, heart disease and diabetes. Another important factor to remember is that medication can play a large contributing factor to developing depression and other mental health conditions.

Losing independence

Seniors who lose their ability to adequately care for themselves on a daily basis are more likely to have mental health setbacks. Chronic pain, poor mobility, and other functional issues might all contribute to an increased risk.

Change in economic status

Many seniors find that retirement necessitates a simpler lifestyle than they're accustomed to, which often necessitates new activities or relocation. If they're handicaps, the effects of those changes may be amplified, requiring even more drastic alterations in their living surroundings.

Loneliness

Due to lack of social interaction. As a result of disabilities, medical issues, the loss of loved ones, and other causes, older persons are more likely to experience feelings of abandonment or isolation. And it's been proven that those feelings have a role in the development of depression and other mental health issues.

Poor dieting

A bad diet can deprive a person of the important nutrients required for a healthy brain and intellect, whether it's by choice, neglect, or financial constraints. A lack of sufficient nourishment can deteriorate a person's mental health over time. Similarly, ingesting alcohol or illicit substances on a frequent basis might produce biological changes that increase the likelihood of having a mental illness.

Family genetics

Genetics may play an influence on a certain individual's mental health. A genetic predisposition to some mental illnesses can be handed down through generations, putting some people at a higher risk than others based solely on their family histories.

Take Heed of Warning Signs

It's not always simple to determine if you or someone you care about is having mental health issues. However, the indications aren't always evident. They might be concealed or unnoticed. That's why knowing what to look out for is crucial. When it comes to seniors and the mental health concerns that may impact them, warning indicators might include:

Feelings of sadness or hopelessness that persist more than a few weeks

Changes in mood, appetite, or energy levels that are unusual

Consistent sleeping problems or oversleeping
Consistent concentration problems

Unrest or a sense of being "on edge"

Reduced capacity to cope with ordinary stress

Irritability, hostility, or fury at an elevated level

High-risk behaviors or acts that frighten others

Worrying excessively about relationships, health, or finances

Obsessive thoughts or obsessive behaviors that interfere with day-to-day life

Emotional numbness

Confusion in familiar situations or repeated memory problems

Alcohol use that is more than usual

Excessive use of prescription medicines

Consistent discomfort, headaches, or digestive problems

Suicidal ideation

These warning signs are serious. The sooner you realize there is a problem, it's imperative to take the proper steps to better your mental health. Yoga is the stepping stone to a better daily route for a healthier mind.

YOGA IS PART OF A NEW LIFESTYLE

Yoga will work best for you when it's beside other lifestyle changes. You are never too old to make this change. Every small change can add to the greater difference in your life. Accompany your yoga practice with activities like:

Eat a balanced diet

Proper nutrition may have a significant impact on your mental health and general vigor. Eat a diverse range of fresh fruits and vegetables, lean and high-quality proteins, healthy fats, whole grains, and calcium-rich meals. Sugar, refined carbohydrates, and excessively processed meals should be avoided wherever feasible.

Maintain healthy sleeping habits

It's a common misconception that elders require less sleep than younger people. Even though the exact quantity varies from person to person, they all require an adequate amount. So, make it a habit to go to bed and wake up at the same hour every day if you can. Consult your doctor if you're having any problems. It's likely that you're suffering from a medical condition such as sleep apnea. It's essential to get adequate sleep in order to maintain excellent mental and physical health.

Mind-Body work

Continue to expand your knowledge. Fill out crossword puzzles or participate in other mind-stimulating exercises or brain teasers.

Take care of medical concerns as soon as possible
Allowing any new physical difficulties to linger for an extended period of time is not a

good idea.

Maintain strong social ties

One of the best strategies to help avoid mental health concerns from interrupting your life is to maintain strong social connections. Accept the help of those who are willing to listen and allow you to express yourself. Friendship and loved ones who are supportive can help you improve your attitude and reduce your stress. They may also be able to assist you with any practical difficulties that influence your quality of life, such as obtaining dependable transportation or budgeting.

Maintain your involvement

Joining a social group or volunteering for a cause you care about might help you feel more connected and fulfilled. Maintaining a sense of community can also help you build self-esteem and become more robust to stress.

Consult your doctor

If you think you could be having a mental health problem, don't hesitate to contact your primary care physician. They may be able to get you started on a treatment plan that will aid in your recovery. They may also be able to connect you with specialist professionals or local mental health services for the elderly and senior population in your area.

Get a second opinion

Because the symptoms of mental health disorders in seniors might differ greatly from those of younger patients, some clinicians have difficulty accurately identifying them. Seniors are also more likely to have several medical illnesses and be on a variety of medications, making identifying mental health difficulties more difficult. So, if possible, get a second opinion from a specialist who works in senior health care or geriatric psychiatry.

Standing your ground

When your mental health is in jeopardy, stand your ground and ignore those who advise you to "suck it up". Try to set your worry of what others might think aside. Allowing their ignorance or bad attitudes to obstruct your therapy and recovery is not a good idea. Also, don't be scared to speak out for your own personal safety and freedom. Nobody has the right to take advantage of your trust or prohibit you from getting help.

Make sure you finish your treatment

Getting healthier doesn't have to be difficult because of your age. Seniors, in fact, may recover from mental health problems equally as well as younger individuals. Take any medications given to you and make every effort to keep all of your therapy and yoga sessions going.

Seek further help

We sometimes require more assistance than our friends and family provide. Never be ashamed to ask. Most towns, thankfully, offer support groups and programs geared at assisting seniors and the elderly with a variety of concerns, including mental health. They may be able to connect you with others who have been in similar situations. Many of them can also provide you free services to aid in your rehabilitation. It's also useful to read a variety of mental health literature, attend local seminars (virtually, if not physically), and look at websites of reputable mental health organizations. You may even want to venture into chair yoga classes around town. It's easier to venture through this journey with other like-minded individuals in your circumstances.

When it comes to your mental health, be proactive. Also, don't be scared to discuss it. It is within your right to do all in your power to be at your best.

Chair Yoga for Weight Loss

Preoccupation with weight control has reached new heights by 2006, according to Yoga Alliance, and the obesity issue continues to approach epidemic proportions.

The number of individuals who are officially classified as obese has reached an all-time high: Approximately 65% of individuals in the United States are overweight, with roughly 30% classified as obese. Being overweight is dangerous because of the problems that come with it, such as an increased risk of heart disease, diabetes, cancer, high blood pressure, and high cholesterol.

People sometimes turn to fad diets or fast fixes to reduce weight, but long-term lifestyle modifications combining reasonable food adjustments and exercise are more likely to promote lifetime weight management.

Normal exercise, even regular mat yoga, is too much for many people with weight problems unless they lose a significant amount of weight. Chair yoga is an excellent workout option for these people. It provides the activity that is so important in a long-term weight-loss regimen. Chair yoga helps to improve muscular tissue, and therefore your metabolic rate. Chair yoga is a stress reliever that also helps you lose weight by reducing stress eating. It also helps to balance the glands and organs, allowing you to better regulate your weight.

Multiple Sclerosis

Multiple Sclerosis (MS) is a central nerve system autoimmune disease, according to experts. Numbness and/or tingling in the limbs, weakness, loss of coordination and/or balance, gait problems, slurred speech, blurred or double vision, bowel and bladder dysfunction, vertigo, and heat intolerance are some of the symptoms.

Despite its popularity, there has only been one high-quality research on yoga with MS patients. The Oregon Health Science University study looked at the effects of yoga and aerobic exercise on cognitive function, tiredness, and mood in 69 volunteers who were randomly allocated to either conventional exercise, yoga, or no exercise. Both individuals who performed yoga and those who did traditional exercise reported less weariness after six months, according to two fatigue measurement tests.

Yoga is a type of medicine that combines the mind, body, and soul. To affect health, it entails a combination of exercise, breathing, and mental attention.

Yoga has a good impact on the brain, which in turn has a positive impact on the immune system, hormones, and involuntary processes like blood pressure and heart rate.

It is a type of exercise as well. For persons with MS, exercise in general is recognized to have various health advantages. Exercise improves muscle tone and cardiovascular health, as well as increasing the synthesis of proteins in the brain (called "growth factors") that drive nerve development, which is particularly important for persons with MS.

Chair yoga is a wonderful option for individuals with MS who find that regular exercise is too difficult. It will help enhance mental alertness, coordination, circulation, energy, flexibility, and general mobility by strengthening their physiology, particularly their neurological system.

Scoliosis

Scoliosis is a spine abnormality characterized by a complicated lateral and rotational curvature. Scoliosis affects 2-3% of the population in the United States, or around 6 million individuals, and there is no treatment. Infants, adolescents, and adults are all affected by scoliosis. Females are eight times more likely than males to reach a treatment required curve magnitude.

This unhealthy curve can worsen over time, resulting in disfigurement, respiratory and digestive issues, and debilitating pain if left unmanaged. The majority of scoliosis patients are diagnosed between the ages of 12 and 16, though the disease affects many adults as well.

Osteoporosis & Osteopenia

Many of you are in situations in your lives that prevent you from exercising. This condition can develop to osteopenia (poor bone mass), which can progress to osteoporosis as we age (a bone disease that makes them more fragile). Chair yoga has been shown to be beneficial in both delaying and reversing these diseases.

If you have osteopenia or osteoporosis, you should avoid any forward bending or trunk contracting postures. Gentle back bending postures that open the chest provide front spine extension, allowing for complete inhalations and exhalations. You'll be able to expel more carbon dioxide, which will help you feel less tired.

The following are some osteoporosis facts provided by FORE (the Foundation for Osteoporosis Research and Education):

At a cost of $17 billion each year, osteoporosis affects 44 million Americans (California's population is about 34 million)

Osteoporosis affects one out of every two women and one out of every eight men at some point in their lives.

People with osteoporosis are more likely to have painful, disfiguring fractures that limit their ability to lead active lifestyles.

According to a recent study, half of all women over 50 have osteoporosis or osteopenia and were unaware of it.

Only 35% of individuals in the United States get the recommended daily calcium intake.

In the United States, an estimated 14 million men have osteopenia or osteoporosis.

Osteoporosis can be treated and even prevented.

People should be aware of their osteoporosis risk and consult their doctors about diagnosis prevention and treatment options.

Arthritis

Arthritis affects the joints, causing pain, stiffness, and swelling. This might make it difficult to do the motions you need to accomplish your job or care for your family on a daily basis.

Those with arthritis who participate in weekly chair yoga practices gain physical strength and mental confidence. You're not required to get up and down from your yoga mat. On the chair, you can get all of the advantages of yoga, including pain and stiffness relief without having to strain yourself getting down to the floor.

Heart Disease

According to Lakshmi Voelker of International Association of Yoga Therapists, the most prevalent cardiovascular illnesses include heart disease and stroke. For both genders, they are the third and first leading causes of death. (Cancer falls somewhere in the middle.) Cardiovascular disease, mostly heart attack or stroke, is responsible for 40% of all fatalities in the United States. In the United States, around 910,000 individuals die each year as a result of cardiovascular disease. This equates to almost one fatality every 35 seconds. It used to be that most of the people were approximately 65 years old or older. Despite this, heart disease and strokes among those aged 15 to 34 have grown. A cardiovascular condition affects 70 million people worldwide. Chair yoga, along with meditation and breathing exercises, can help manage heart problems.

Diabetes

Diabetes affects 20.8 million children and adults in the United States, accounting for 7% of the population. Despite the fact that 14.6 million individuals have been diagnosed with diabetes, 6.2 million people (almost one-third) remain ignorant of their condition.

By doing chair yoga for 40 minutes everyday, you can lower your fasting blood sugar levels. When type 11 diabetics do chair yoga on a regular basis, their lung capacity improves by 10%, and their blood sugar management and pulmonary functions improve with time (Voelker, 2021).

Supplement to Cancer Therapy

Yoga has lately gained popularity as an alternative cancer treatment. The medical community recognized yoga's advantages (such as flexibility, strength, improved range of motion, and relaxation) in the treatment of cancer symptoms and side effects. Yoga has been proven to alleviate stress related to cancer therapies and/or disease progression, which supports the concept that it might enhance a cancer patient's quality of life.

The Memorial Sloan-Kettering, the MD Anderson Cancer Center, and the Dana-Farber Cancer Institute have all taken efforts to provide yoga as an alternate adjunct therapy for cancer patients.

Yoga and its advantages for cancer patients have been studied using a number of criteria including cancer kinds, stages of disease, and treatment levels. Improved sleep quality, decreased sadness, reduced stress and anxiety, less cancer-related discomfort, physiological benefits, less pain, and an overall higher quality of life are among the findings. Depending on the kind and stage of cancer, as well as when the patient begins yoga treatments, patients report varying degrees of recovery.

Lungs

The fact that one-third of all fatalities are caused by lung illnesses can be attributed in part to shallow breathing. Some people only breathe through their upper lungs, while others only breathe through their diaphragm (power part). Only a few people are able to fully breathe. Secretions build up in the regions of the lungs that aren't utilized, and the tissues become devitalized.

Yoga's science of the breath, Pranayama, can help those with breathing difficulties. Pranayama is a set of practices for expanding the capacity of your lungs. Pranayama also aids in the regulation of the temperature of the breath flow, which helps to alleviate a variety of lung-related issues.

With just 30 minutes of chair yoga, you may ease lung issues by relaxing neck muscles and improving posture while sitting.

Disabled People

According to data published by the United States Census Bureau, 18% (51.2 million) of Americans had a disability in 2002, and 12% (32.5 million) had a severe impairment with 4 million being children aged 6 to 14.

According to the National Council for Support of Disability Issues (NCSD), for those with impairments, exercise is essential. It boosts your self-esteem and motivates you to strive for perfection in your disability in your own unique way.

With weekly chair yoga sessions, disabled persons who are wheelchair confined begin to appreciate life and become more joyful.

On the wheelchair, turning your yoga practice into an enjoyable breathing and movement activity has shown to be beneficial. Your confidence grows, and you'll want to conduct habitual sessions as time goes on.

Contraindications

A contraindication is a condition that makes participating in a certain activity more dangerous. If you have a significant physical or mental condition, consult with a healthcare expert before beginning chair yoga.

Over the years, we have gathered a long list of contraindications to chair yoga for a variety of illnesses. If you have balance or other physical difficulties, remember that yoga on a chair provides a better overall atmosphere. This boosts self-assurance, resulting in increased inner and exterior strength.

Chair yoga is beneficial for seniors. Use this book as a guide through your new journey. It is said that exercise is the best medicine. Chair yoga is an effective and enjoyable exercise suited for seniors. Once you begin your poses, you will feel relaxation flowing through your body. Even 10 minutes a day, or night, can make a difference. Explore these poses at your own pace. Embrace deep breathing and meditation as part of the routine. With this gentle form of yoga, you will experience improvement in your health. Let peace enter your body and mind. Let go of tension and welcome tranquility. Take control of your well-being one pose at a time.

Namaste.